Welcome to your lifestyle refresh! I'm so glad you have taken the initiative to transform your life much like I did mine back that cold December Day in 2017. Frankley I'll be honest for this to work you must be willing to commit to 30 min a day of personal growth and development. If you're not willing to invest in yourself and your future by making a 30 minute commitment you may want to evaluate your current priorities and if you still cannot commit then this book will be here when you are ready.

To explain the purpose of a lifestyle refresh I want to take a moment to point out what a lifestyle refresh is not; this is not just a weightloss plan, this is not really a diet, this is not a competition or slim down quick process. This program is designed to help coach and offer direction to help you create a healthier happier lifestyle designed specifically for you and your life. There are no daily meal plans. Because I believe our lives are better lived if we are in control of our own choices. We have 1 life to live and I don't believe we can live our happiest life living in a box of rules someone else designed for themselves. While we are all different and live vastly different lifestyles I believe everyone should find value in this program regardless of your specific goals.

Now for the Program Rules:
- Before beginning any diet or exercise program please consult with your Dr. This is not a diet or exercise program.
- No negativity. No complaining. No excuses.
-Keep an open mind and take your time to complete the weekly units to make the most of this.

Unit 1.

Start Small. Picture this someone approaches you and 2 friends and tells you if you can run or walk 100 miles in 24 hours they'll give you 1 million dollars. Your first friend looks at you and says I can't even run a mile. I am out! They simply choose not to play the game. They didn't believe the reward was worth the effort. They didn't have the right mindset. Now your second friend takes off sprinting assuming the first to get to 100 miles will earn the million dollars. After 25 miles he develops terrible blisters and shortly after must give up the opportunity. They wanted to be in the game but burnt out too quickly to finish. He gave up after a set back. But you... You really want that million dollars you don't actually know if you can go 100 miles in 24 hrs but you're gonna give it a shot. So you start jogging and keep jogging. While jogging you start thinking. You start forming a plan. You do the math. You figure out if I can go a little over 4 miles every hour for 24 hrs you could possibly do this. Now will you make it 100 miles in that 24 hrs? The only way to really know is to give it a shot. Maybe you made it the first time. Maybe you fail but the stranger never said you had to do it in the first 24 hrs. Maybe you keep practicing and training and one day you make it 100 miles in 24 hrs and are awarded your prize. Regardless of the outcome the only players in the game are the ones choosing to participate. If you're not in the game. You can't "win".

The definition of change is to "make or become different". In life we have the choice to change. Everyday we wake up in this country with lots of choices to make. Many days we make the same choices. These choices add up over time. Right now we are living the results of the actions and choices we previously made. If we want our lives to change and become different we must make our actions and choices be different.

Another definition of change is 'to take or use instead of" Right now we are using a lot of the same daily choices. To change our lives we must use new choices instead of the old ones.

Take some time today to identify 4 choices you're making that are not bringing you the desired results you want or you feel you want to change to improve your life. Why are you making these unsatisfactory choices in the first place? What can you do to help yourself not make that same choice in the future. This isn't always a simple open and shut case. What you may originally identify as a late night snacking habit that you want to change may actually end up being identified as an emotional eating situation later on. The only way to know is to start somewhere. Be honest with yourself. Don't think negatively. Don't assume because you failed to change in the past means you'll fail again. Don't take yourself out of the game on the first day! If you feel comfortable, share below!

Now for the hard part. I only want you to pick 1 to work on this week. ONLY 1. It's tempting to try and work on all of them at once but that can leave us feeling overwhelmed and uncomfortable. Too many changes in the first 20 miles and we will end up burnt out, exhausted and unable to finish the game. Remember to tackle this thing 1 mile at a time!

Unit 2

H20! GATORADE! H20! GATORADE! While many people laughed at a certain waterboy, he knew the importance of staying hydrated. After all his Alaskan Glacier Water saved the day and helped his team win the Bourbon Bowl!

Water helps our bodies absorb nutrients, regulate body temperature, flush out toxins and waste and helps prevent constipation. Yet many of us are chronically dehydrated. Which can lead to constant fatigue ongoing muscle weakness frequent headaches and dry or flaky skin

Today's challenge is to think about water weight in a new way. Oftentimes we are upset the scale goes up when we start properly hydrating and get discouraged. But after our bodies become properly hydrated we are healthier and it can help us reach our long term better health goals faster. When the scale goes up because we are hydrating properly that's a good gain not a bad one. So the next time the scale goes up due to proper hydration think to yourself about all the good reasons for that gain. Here's 10 reasons why you should want to drink more water -75% of your brain

-regulates body temp -keeps skin looking healthy -helps burn fat -prevents constipation -decrease fatigue -carries oxygen to cells -helps flush out toxins -best no calorie beverage

Today's challenge is to research pee color charts and identify where you are on the chart range. begin working towards getting your pee color into the preferred chart color range. Track your water consumption today and see just how much water you really are drinking in a day. Only about 1/5th of our daily water consumption comes from foods so the rest we should be drinking.

Unit 3

The motivation myth. A common misconception is that motivation will come and go but most successful people know that motivation doesn't magically show up to help us get started or continue on our journeys. Motivation comes from a feeling of accomplishment brought on by results that came from taking action. Think of the last time you felt "motivated"? What else was going on in your life at that time. How did you feel? What did you do with your "motivation"? Oftentimes this "motivation" is when we are already making some good choices that are bringing us closer to our goals. Luckily we can drum up a little motivation ourselves by taking simple steps even when we don't "feel it".

This week try writing down 3 things you want to accomplish everyday and physically mark off each of the 3 things as you do them. Make sure you physically write them down and leave them where you can see them. Mentally we receive a greater reward by visually seeing ourselves complete tasks and watching our to do list get smaller leaves us feeling accomplished and productive. When you finish, take a moment to look at your list. How do you feel? If you did not complete your list try again tomorrow setting smaller tasks that you can more easily accomplish until you've built up your self confidence and can add even more to your to do list. Now that you've completed your to do list do you feel like you can accomplish even more tomorrow? Continue to use these 3 items to do lists daily. Not all need to be chore or work related. Try adding in a few to do your looking forward to daily like 30 min of reading a book on your lunch break or call or textinging an old friend. Mix it up and make sure your to dos are something you don't normally do during the day like brushing your teeth. These should be tasks that are helping to move you forward in different areas of your lifestyle change,

Unit 4

Excuses

In our journeys we can choose to be 1 of 2 people. The I CANT person or the I CAN person. Obviously we will never start our journey or not get far if we are the I CANT person. Back a few years ago I was very much an I CANT person. I would often tell myself I CAN'T lose weight because I can't go to the gym. Or I CAN'T afford to eat healthy. Or I CAN'T workout.

Truthfully the only difference between an I CANT person and an I CAN person is the next step. An I CAN person may see something they CAN'T do right now but they look for what they CAN do instead. EXAMPLE: I can't go to the gym because I have a daughter no daycare can't afford it or any other excuse you want to enter here now an I CANT person stops right here and blames this reason for their lack of progress but an I CAN person asks themselves what they could do instead that would help them get the same or similar results. I CAN'T go to the gym but I CAN do at home workouts. I CAN go for a walk. I CAN do seated shadow boxing. I CAN clean vigorously. I CAN do a lot of things to be active and moving and get similar results as those that CAN go to the gym.

Today's challenge is to help you start switching that mindset. Ask yourself, is there something you recently told yourself you couldn't do and gave up on? Find 3 excuses that you feel are holding you back from hitting your goals in life and then list 3 things you can do instead.

Here's some examples that are not fitness related: I CAN'T get a second job out of the home because child care is too expensive but I CAN look for at home work opportunities.

I can't go to church because I have to work on Sundays but I can listen to radio programs or sermon replays online

When we remove the option for excuses we discover we are in fact in control of our lives. Just because you can't do something today doesn't mean you should completely give up on our goals. We can still make progress as long as we are still actively making choices and taking action to get there.

Unit 5

Calorie Density

Calorie Density is a measure of the **calorie** content of food relative to its weight or volume. It is also called energy **density** and is usually measured as **calories** per 3.5 ounces (100 grams) of food. Choosing foods with a low **calorie density** can help with weight loss.

A grape and raisin. Same thing one is just processed more than the other. Which do you think is more calorie dense? Which will fill you up more?

Today I want you to look at 5 of your favorite foods and calculate their calorie densities. Are you choosing low calorie dense foods to fill you up like green leafy veggies and water filled fruits or more calorie dense foods like nuts and other boxed processed foods.

As a food addict calorie counting actually hurt my attempts at weight loss because it felt restrictive and oftentimes we underestimate how much we are eating unless we cook, measure and track every single item we eat. When I started my lifestyle change I didn't want to have to put that much time and attention into food every single day for the rest of my life so I choose to keep calorie density in mind when making my food choices. I was still mindful of what I was eating and how much but I felt good about my choices and more full when I ate low calorie dense foods and was able to lose weight while fueling my body with plenty of food and never hungry.

Unit 6

Count Colors not Calories

Yesterday we talked about Calorie Density and how I used that information on my journey to make better choices to fuel my body without overdoing it on calories and needing to track and measure all our food. Today I want to talk about colors and food.

Natural foods come in so many different colors and each food (and color) has something beneficial for us in it. Today I want you to pick a color of food and research what benefits are associated with that color and food item. EXAMPLE: Carrots - Orange- **beta-Carotene-**Eye Sight. Find out what colors you feel you should be focused on adding into your diet.

Often I'll look at what I'm eating and ask myself how I can make this healthier. Most times the answer is...add more veggies! An example I often share is I used to love steak and cheese subs. However those weren't the best choices to make when trying to lose weight so I asked myself how can I make a steak and cheese healthier??? The answer was in green peppers. By removing the bread and adding a green pepper as the serving vehicle I cut hundreds of calories and was still able to enjoy my steak and cheese in moderation while adding flavor and more vitamins and antioxidants for my health.

Unit 7
Give yourself Permission. A Lot of times we are so focused on the cants, the I have tos, and the musts of our programs or plans we dont leave ourselves any wiggle room. Is anyone claustrophobic? When you start building walls around yourself things start to seem smaller and cramped and you feel too big. Today I want you to give yourself permission to enjoy life. Give yourself permission to enjoy things in moderation. BUT here's the challenge: identify several of the opportunity costs of enjoying that thing.
What is an opportunity cost? It's what you give up when you make a choice. So the opportunity cost of brushing your teeth daily? You're giving up additional cavities. Your giving up morning breath. You're giving up additional plaque build up.

So give yourself permission to enjoy a treat today but first think of 5 things you're giving up by choosing to indulge. For me my indulgences are sweet treats so I have to ask myself am I willing to give up clearer skin for this because sugar makes me break out. Am I willing to give up that healthy good choice feeling I am enjoying today. Am I willing to give up these 500 calories that are part of 3200 that are a part of a 1lb deficit to enjoy this treat? Am I willing to give up a clearer mind and balanced blood sugar to enjoy this treat.

Sometimes the treat is worth it. I don't often eat flour products but if I was vacationing in France and had the opportunity to enjoy some amazing authentic french treats I would. But if I'm just in the supermarket and see a box of snack cakes it's not going to be worth the opportunity cost to me.

If you have gout attacks it's a lot easier to make the choice to skip the all you can eat shrimp buffett if you know it's going to cause a gout attack. The opportunity cost of not having a gout attack is just too high to give up for just 1 meal.

Now for the fun part:

If you choose to indulge, how do you feel about your choice? What made it worth it to you?

If you choose to skip the treat how do you feel about your choice? What made it worth it to skip it to you?

Bonus Activity:
Next time you're presented with the choice to indulge or not repeat the same process but ask yourself is there a healthier choice I could enjoy later if I skip this treat right now.

Often when Macyn wants Ice Cream I'll skip it and choose to enjoy a vanilla greek yogurt banana and berry treat instead. I put it in a fancy glass and decorate it with almond slivers and drizzle of honey. It makes me feel fancy and is fun to make so it makes the choice to skip the banana split easier and more enjoyable

Unit 8

Momentum: the impetus gained by a moving object
Impetus: the force that makes something happen or happen more quickly.

We've all heard the term momentum. Watching football we know which team has the momentum. In sales we talk about salesmen using the momentum to finish the month strong. When we have the momentum things are happening but wait how did we get that momentum in the first place? By doing something. By taking an action and that action paid off by bringing us closer to our goals. So if we're doing something and it's working we're going to keep doing it because it's working for us. But for us to get momentum we have to actively take those first few steps. We DON'T know if those first steps are going to work. We don't know if the quarterback is going to connect with a receiver down field but if he never threw the ball the receiver couldn't catch it. Sometimes the quarterback could throw a perfect pass and it not get caught. So no momentum was gained. Does that mean we punt on 2nd down? No, we keep playing, keep passing and sometimes we change things up to see if maybe a run game is a better approach against this defense.

Like in the game of football there's going to be challenges that get in the way of our goals. Not every week are we going to score a touchdown or a loss of weight. You will win some and you will lose some.

This week's challenge: Break the year up into 4 quarters. How many weeks are in each quarter? Now picture where you want to be in a year. Write it down or share it here if you'd like. To reach that goal break it down into 4 steps or phases going into the year. Now commit to your plan for at least 1 full quarter of the year. That's 3 months out of 12. If what approach you are taking does not create momentum in 3 months it may be time for a new approach or to tweak your game plans. But today we are setting a Specific Goal for ourselves to complete within the year writing it down and committing to a plan to get started on working towards that goal.

Unit 9

Measuring Success:
Yesterday's Challenge was to write down a yearly goal for yourself. How many physically wrote it down like I requested? Be honest, if not with me, with yourself. Because honestly you have almost double the chance of reaching your goals simply by writing them down. If one cannot be bothered to write down a goal how important is it to you anyway?
According to Forbes men are more likely to write down goals then women. Why do you think that is? Are men better at writing? Doubtful. I believe the answer lies in social stigmas but regardless of the answer the statistics show if you want to reach your goals you need to write them down for 2 reasons: external storage and encoding. External storage is easy. you're storing the information contained in your goal in a location (e.g. a piece of paper) that is very easy to access and review at any time. You could post that paper anywhere in your office or home. It doesn't take a scientist to know you will remember something much better if you're staring at it every single day.

But there's a deeper phenomenon within writing down goals: encoding. Encoding is the biological process by which the things we perceive travel to our brain's hippocampus where they're analyzed. From there, decisions are made about what gets stored in our long-term memory and, in turn, what gets discarded. Writing improves that encoding process. In other words, when you write it down it has a much greater chance of being remembered.

So todays challenge is to write down your short: 1 month-3 month medium: 1 year -3 years and long term goals: 3+ years goals: in the S.M.A.R.T. format: Specific, Measurable, Attainable, Realistic, Time frame. If you aren't familiar with the S.M.A.R.T technique a quick google search can help!

Unit 10:

Measuring success part 2:

So now we know how to set goals and reasonable time frames for us to work towards goals and when to know when a game plan change may be necessary but today let's look at what success really means to us as humans. A very specific goal. We set them all the time but what happens when we fail to reach a goal? Are we just losers and worthless? No, not at all. To me people that set their goals just out of reach are always going to get themselves further then the person who sets their goals so low they never have to try.

Failure of a goal isn't always a bad thing. If your goal is to raise 10k for your charity and you turn in $9,000 do you think the people benefiting from your fundraising are going to laugh at you for falling short? No so why do we beat ourselves up over just missing an advantageous goal? Take the fear out of failure. Most of us were raised to win. The winner gets the prize in sports, the winner gets the job, the girl the money in any movie you watch. But your lifes not a movie. its not a competition. its what you make it! A person who sets huge enormous goals and sometimes falls just short is going to live a much more fulfilling life than the person who never sets a goal because they never believed in themselves enough to try and let their fears control their life rather than taking the wheel themselves to direct themselves where they wanted to go. Fear of Failure is very real in all of us but so is courage. When it comes to setting advantageous goals for ourselves you don't need to be scared, find that courage to chase dreams that matter to you. Don't be a passenger on the ship of life because you're afraid of being the captain and getting lost. Take control of what is yours to control in life...yourself.

Today's Challenge: Identify what areas in life your letting fear control you in. What are the consequences of failure to hit the goals you would have set for yourself if you weren't afraid to take control. What would you gain if you were able to reach those goals? Do you think you could take smaller steps towards reaching that goal with less risk? How does that sense of fear make you feel about yourself?

Unit 11:

Treating yourself like a friend:

I'm fat. I'm ugly. I'm disgusting. I hate myself. I am stupid. I can't do anything right. I'm an idiot.

How many of us have said these things to ourselves?

How many of us use these phrases?

You're fat. You are ugly. You are disgusting. I hate you. You are stupid. You can't do anything right. You are an idiot?

How many of us have said these phrases to our friends and meant them?

My guess is most of us won't admit to talking to our friends like that and if we do we probably don't have many friends.

In school we are taught to be kind to others at an early age but how many of us were taught to be kind to ourselves?

People tell me all the time they don't know how to love themselves. Self love starts with self respect. If someone talked to me like that I wouldn't respect them. I wouldn't want to be their friend and I wouldn't want to do anything to help them out. So why do we think it's ok for us to treat ourselves worse than we treat others?

Today's Challenge is to start looking at yourself as a person. Obviously you are a person but I want you to step outside yourself for a moment. Think about the thoughts going through your head. Are they kind? Are they respectful? Are they positive? Are they productive?

Today when you talk negatively to yourself stop. Don't say something to yourself that you wouldn't say to others. We need to be open to constructive criticism. We can't be perfect and shouldn't believe we are but we don't need to be a bully either. If you need to do better at something tell yourself that and move on. To build self love we first need to work on self respect. If you don't respect yourself you can't love yourself.

Our brains are wired to think negatively most of us have been using negative self talk all our lives. It's not something that is going to switch in a day or two but something you need to be working on every single day like in a relationship if we don't practice and show love and respect to our partners we will lose it.

Unit 12:

Benefits of whole foods

What was the last meal you ate? How much of it was grown exactly as you ate it? Very rarely do we eat foods that havent been processed. Most of it is at least cleaned and cut. Usually we cook it or steam it or bake it. All of that is a means of processing. But how much processing is too much processing? We all have a different answer for that. To me natural foods don't have chemicals added into the food itself I don't eat a lot of flour based products or grains or foods that have been bleached. What's right and reasonable for me and for you can be different and that's ok but what today's unit is on is the benefits of adding more whole foods:

Low in sugar (even fruits are lower in sugar then most processed foods)
High in nutrients - bleaching and the stripping of nutrients just happens in processed foods
High in fiber
Better Balances your Blood Sugar
Good for your skin
More variety
May prevent overeating
Better for dental health
Removes the focus on dieting

Because this is a lifestyle refresh im not going to go in the scientific detail behind each but today's challenge is to research whole foods and 3 benefits of eating more natural

Unit 13:

One of the most common excuses of why people don't eat healthier is they can't afford it. I'm here to break that myth. Eating convenient natural foods is expensive. Whole foods from the grocery store can save you time and money when done correctly.

Today's challenge is to join a facebook support group that offers recipes and advice on eating clean and cheap. Or look for cheap healthy eating blogs online. I've found several myself just from a quick search on cheap healthy meals or eating healthy on a budget. Then come back and write down a few good tips you've found

Unit 14:
 (13 continued)

As most of you may have discovered meal prep and planning is a great way to help save money when making healthier food choices. I used to just buy random things at the grocery store and a lot of my produce went to waste because I didn't know what to do with it. Why make a salad when I can just throw a microwave meal in and be eating 3 min later?

 Meal prep and planning does take time to get used to and I would never advise someone just jump in with all 3 meals and 2 snacks a day planned out everyday for the rest of your life. But today I want you to think of a way you can begin to incorporate meal planning into your life gradually.

Maybe start with boiling hard boiled eggs for breakfast for the week. Or try planning your lunches during the work week ahead of time. Start with planning 1 meal a day for a certain number of days and see how you like it.

Meal Prep doesn't mean you have to eat the same things every day forever. Maybe you make one big lunch to split up for the work week and then switch it up next week. Or maybe meal prep to you looks more like saving food from dinner for lunch tomorrow. We all are going to have a different starting spot here but the theme and message is the same for everyone. If we fail to plan we fail to plan.

Today's Challenge is to set a plan of attack for meal prep.

Unit 15:

Try something new!

I love this one. We get so sucked into the monotony of day to day life many of us forget to really live! New things excite us and add new colors and flavors to our lives. How many new things have you tried recently? Did you regret ever trying something new?

I tried a new job once and it failed miserably but it taught me alot about myself and the company that I hadn't known before. It was eye opening and stressful but it was worth the experience and the knowledge I learned.

New recipes can add new variety to our meals or flop fenominaly

New workouts can excite and invigorate or remind you of weaknesses you need to work

New walking routes can create a change of scenery or open a world of new friends

Learning a new language can increase your value in the workforce

A new hobby just might be what you need to get excited about life again and give you something to look forward to

Today's challenge is to try something new this week. Plan it today, put it on your calendar and make sure you do it!

Unit 16:

Exercise

I used to hate this word. It used to bring me a lot of anxiety and remind me of just how far I'd let myself go. I could barely walk to my car. I was too lazy to put on shoes in the morning because I would get breathless just bending over to put them on.

So instead of focusing on forcing myself to do things I didn't want to do I asked myself what I was willing to do to be active. At first it was cleaning or maybe a 7 min youtube video on standing ab exercises. Then I tried yoga and fell in love. I could literally roll out of bed as is and start stretching and moving my body slowly but purposefully. I found out truvision had a 10k challenge where I could earn free products and swag by hitting 10k steps a day so that motivated me to start walking. I wasn't able to hit that target or even get close to it in the beginning. But I kept walking on my lunch breaks and trying to go further and longer over time.

Because I never forced myself to do one thing I've had the opportunity to try many things. The only exercise rule I've set for myself is I won't go to bed until I've done 10 min of purposeful activity a day. The rest has just been a natural progression. I keep doing more because I enjoy what I'm doing.

They say to try new things 3 times, once to get over the fear of doing it twice to learn how to do it and a third time to figure out whether you like it or not. Back in college I tried yoga and HATED it. Like literally cursed the name yoga. I'd rather have been in 12 mauls in a rugby match then spend 15 min on a yoga mat. It just wasn't for me at the time. So make sure you don't miss out because you are keeping a closed mine and not retrying things you have in the past.

Today's challenge is to look into purposeful movement activities you might enjoy and can do safely but have never tried or haven't retried in over 5 years. Maybe it's seated shadow boxing if you have mobility issues. Maybe you've always wanted to try body groove or zumba. Maybe you wanna try a power clean session on your home while rocking some 80s rock. Look on youtube for free workouts that you might enjoy and schedule a time to give them a try this week ! You choose! It's your life!

Unit 17:

The Power of Positivity

We all hear it, we all see it but do we really believe it? I was a skeptic HUGE skeptic. I had a boss that used to tell me positive thoughts brought positive results. I just thought he was tired of people complaining. Never really "bought into" the idea.

Turns out there's actually truth in this. As in actual behavioral change science. Yeah. Science. Sciency Science. Like real science. Look it up!

Our brains only have so much room so if we allow too much negative in then there's not as much room for the positive. If we constantly are focused on negatives that's what we are going to look for and see. If we constantly are focused on being a positive person then we are going to recognize and seek more positive.

Today's challenge is to look for the positives in your life. If you've been in a negative mindset for a while this will be more challenging for you then others and will take a lot of practice. It takes active work. Everyday because our brains are wired to look for the negatives out of survival instincts.

But just like a computer we can work to reprogram our brains to work towards our goals and not against them.

When something bad happens today don't look at it as a negative try and put a positive swing on things. You drop an ice cream cone oh well you didn't need the calories anyway and the floor needed cleaned too. You make a mistake now you learned something. Today I want you to be so overly positively positive that you cant stand yourself.

I learn a lot from rereading children's books with Macyn. One that sticks out to me is a book about a family of bears. In one of the books in the series the family forgets their manners so the Momma Bear makes a chart of punishments for typical poor manners. The cubs worried about the chore chart devise a plan to be so overly polite that momma will call the whole thing off. Only she doesn't because over time the cubs forget to be so overly polite they just become polite and the Papa Bear is the only one left doing the chores.

So today let's try being overly positive ! See if it has an impact on anyone else around you. Did anyone notice? How did you feel? A little silly? A little happy? Maybe truly a little more positive?

Unit 18:
After yesterday's parade of positivity lets bring things back to a more sober topic. ACE Factors.

If you've never heard of an ACE factor before I would like for you to do some research on the impacts of Adverse Childhood Experiences. There is a great test you can take on NPRs website https://www.npr.org/sections/health-shots/2015/03/02/387007941/take-the-ace-quiz-and-learn-what-it-does-and-doesnt-mean

Before reading up on ACES were you aware that your childhood would affect your health later on in life? How do you feel after reading up on ACE factors? Do you feel like maybe some of your current health issues or lifestyle choices are impacted by your own childhood?

There is no way one person can really learn, absorb and use all the information on ACE factors in a day so please don't feel like you need to tackle any of this in a single day. It can take some people years to fully understand and develop a plan to work through much of the mental trauma some of us have been exposed to especially if your ACE factors are over 3 .

Unit 19:

Marketing!

Just what you thought you'd find in a lifestyle refresh right? But knowledge is power when we know how we are being marketed so we can identify it and use our knowledge to help us avoid the pitfalls that were designed to cause us to buy more food or certain types of food.

Often restaurants use the colors red and yellow because we eat more when we're visually surrounded by those colors. Blue and green put us more at ease but when we're at ease we tend to think less about budgets and spend more.

What colors do your favorite stores/restaurants incorporate in their decor and branding? Have you ever consciously asked yourself if your visual cues are being played on to encourage consumption of more? What colors are in your own home? Do you think they use any other senses to subconsciously encourage you to buy more? Hearing? Smell? Touch? There's a reason car dealers allow you to touch and drive a new car because it's harder to say no once you've physically sat behind that seat. Ever hear music or calming sounds while shopping? Aroma plays a strong role in restaurants ever walked out of somewhere and smelt something that "reminded" you that you're hungry?

Tobacco Marketing Gurus were forced to give up cartoon characters and other characters that came off as cool or fun because it encouraged people to smoke. So they used what they knew about marketing tobacco in the processed food industry instead what was once camels and cowboys smoking are now rabbits, leprechauns, birds, tigers and sports athletes telling us what to eat on TV as well as on the boxes themselves.

Grocery stores have always had sugary products at eye level for children because they know sugar is addictive. Kids love sugar. Parents Hate Tantrums. That one is not hard to figure out. Kids love colors and there's a whole rainbow of them waiting at checkout areas full of candy and sweets and other snacks. Remember an addict is a customer for the rest of their lives.

I'm not going to preach on this too much but instead ask you to do your own research today. What ways have you been unknowingly influenced to buy or buy more somewhere without even realizing it. What other ways do you think marketers target people to encourage more spending?

Unit 20:

Counting vs Accountability

Who here has heard of calorie counting? Who here knows they need a calorie deficit to lose weight? Who here loves weighing measuring fixing all of their own food for the rest of their lives so they can manage their weight? *crickets* Not me!

Counting calories or using a point system is a great way to lose weight but who wants to live like that for the rest of their lives? I'm a busy mom. I ain't got time for that.

Serving sizes are important, yes. Knowing calorie amounts of food is important, yes. BUT here's the thing we don't need to take it down to an exact science for tracking to be effective.

You see simply writing down what we eat is just as effective in keeping people accountable. No one wants to write down they ate an entire pizza themselves. Have I done it? yes. Was I tracking my food consumption then no. 4 slices ehhh I've probably wrote that down a few times. BUT typically most people know if they have to write this down on paper they are going to be more accountable with what and how much they are eating.

I am so lazy though that I don't even want to do that in life but I did. I did track not calories or points but when I'm struggling to maintain or cut I do write down what I eat. It provides accountability and a record for myself to go back and review how I could change my lifestyle and what I'm eating to help me better reach my nutrition goals. If someones working out more they may just be interested in making sure they are adding in more protein.

Once you've tracked for a while it becomes automatic and routine. We are creatures of habit. Taco Tuesday anyone? We fix a lot of the same meals over and over occasionally trying new things which is great for us that don't want to have to track calorie count or add up points.

Today's challenge is to begin keeping a food journal if you don't already could be electronic and could be paper in pencil. Write down what you ate and roughly how much you ate. Examples could be a bag of chips or handful of grapes you

don't have to be exact here. Actually I don't want it to be. I want it easy and simple. For those using apps that count calories do your best to ignore them at least for a week.
Do you feel like writing your food down keeps you accountable? For those that calorie count or point count were you able to have success without tracking to exact details? How accurate do you think your calorie counting really is? Did you add in high calorie condiments and add ons like ketchup sour cream, other sauces and oils you used to cook with as well as beverages?

Unit 21:
Stop Quitting

Easier said than done right? Why do people quit? They don't enjoy what they are doing. They don't feel the rewards are worth the work. They feel like they can't reach their end goal. Or they feel there's a better way to get what they want.

I can't say why you quit in the past. I can't tell you that you wont quit in the future. But I can tell you that you can change your mindset if you want to.

We don't quit on things we love. We don't quit when the rewards are worth the effort. We don't quit when we know we are almost there. We don't quit when we know the shortest distance between what we want and where we are is right in front of us.

Make sure your goals are in front of you. Make sure your are doing things you love. Make sure you are giving yourself time for rest and relaxation so you don't suffer burn out. Make sure you know what you are doing is moving forward 1 step at a time. I can't tell you how long it will take you to reach your goal but I can tell you that you won't reach the goal if you stop chasing it. Time is going to pass whether we put the work in or not. It's up to you to decide if you want to spend your time working for what you want or starting and stopping over and over again.

Take a break if you must. Try a new approach if you want. But don't quit.

Today's challenge is to share a story of a successful person who didn't quit that inspires you. Most successful people have a story. A real down and dirty tear jerker. Rarely do great people come from mediocre and uneventful lives. Rock bottom has built more successful people then privilege ever has. Because people who live and stay in their comfort zone don't grow. Sure there are wealthy individuals born into privilege but is wealth our only measure of success. If it was given to you is it really yours? Who is someone who really inspires you and what's their story?

Some of my favorite success stories are
Oprah (if you are known by your first name alone you know your successful)
Steve Harvey &
Audrey Hepburn (did you know she had to eat tulips to survive as a child)

Unit 22

Atomic Habits

Atomic habits are something you do every day without even thinking about it. If you were raised to brush your teeth everyday you probably do it and don't even think about it. Maybe you've developed the same atomic habit as I of reaching to check your phone as soon as you wake up.

We don't think about atomic habits, we just do them and if we don't it bothers us. If we do the same things day after day it becomes a habit. If we do it for longer periods of time it becomes an atomic habit.

Today's challenge is to identify one of your "bad" atomic habits and try to not do it today and pick 1 habit to work to build into an atomic one. You may forget because it's so ingrained into your lifestyle today so just continue to put it on your do list until you're able to skip that bad habit and start building that new good one. Maybe you have a bad habit of checking facebook as soon as you get to the office. Or maybe you have a bad habit of checking your phone at the dinner table. Pick one habit you think would make your life better if you didn't do it and one that would be better if you did if possible try to replace a bad one with a good one. Say for example you check facebook as soon as you get to the office let's switch it for a good one like saying hello or checking in on your coworkers. Maybe you have a bad habit of reaching for a soda in the fridge for lunch and you switch it with having a full bottle of water with your lunch. It's up to you it's your life! You can start off with easy habits and work your way up to harder ones if you'd like or jump right in and tackle the big ones first then work on the little as you go.

Unit 23:

Ditch the diet

I'm not talking about ditching Drs. orders here so if you have medical advice on what is right for you to eat then please do that! BUT if your one of the people like me who sees a shiny new fad diet and jumps on board to see if it works for you too I'm here to share a few things I've learned with you

1. Most social media fad diet accounts are fake. Reach out to them, talk to them. Ask for specifics. Really dig in to see if its a real person with a real story or if its a weight loss success story catfish. I try to respond to as many people as I can and post daily life videos. My friends and family all know I'm real but still get called a fake and a scam daily. So lets us a little skepticism on these new success stories as well before we jump right in.

2. Someone else designed that diet for themselves. So the creator of keto was ok with never eating fruit again...I'm not. That sounds like a really restrictive life to live.

3. Mail order meals...again i'm sure it could work for you but do you really want to eat food from your mailbox for the rest of your life. Having someone else cook for you and plan your meals sounds great but what happens when you stop ordering them. Will YOU be able to maintain that lifestyle?

4. Workouts Programs. While not necessarily a scam or bad thing just remember not all workouts are built for everyone. Some will require you to modify or just not be something that is enjoyable for you. Some people like me cannot stand to admit I just can't do that yet and end up causing themselves

injury by pushing too far. If a workout isn't for you or isn't for you right now doesn't mean it's not effective for someone else but we aren't trying to cram ourselves into someone else's version of a healthy happy life we are trying to build our own. Plus abs are built in the kitchen not the gym!

Unit 24:

Learn to Cook

Some of you might be excellent at this already but some of us are probably like me. The fanciest thing I made before I met Mike was probably grilled cheese. On my lifestyle transformation I actually made a swap that worked out really well. We traded eating out for date nights with several meal prep services. We would order 2 meals a week and they come with food recipe cards and instructions. It was so fun and I learned a ton! Mike actually started letting me cook for a while as an italian male that was hard for him lol The more I practiced the better I got. Pretty soon I felt confident enough to start on other recipes I found online that I wanted to try that looked great and incorporated more of the healthy foods that I was interested in. (who doesn't have a 100 saved recipes they've never made)

Today's Challenge is to find a new recipe for you to try this week. Pick a healthy one please! It doesn't have to be fancy or hard but be something new and exciting that you're looking forward to making. If it doesn't work out no worries you gave it a shot, pick another one and give it another go a different week or will help you identify what areas of weakness you have in the kitchen. If it does then you've found another great dish you can add to your favorites list!

Unit 25

Set Boundaries

Often in life we find ourselves pushing ourselves too far. We need healthy boundaries in relationships, in real estate, in schools, everywhere. While the definition of a boundary is a line that limits that doesn't mean we have to view our boundaries in a negative light. Our boundaries should offer us a freedom in life while protecting us from harm either from others or ourselves.

We caution teens against relationships without boundaries because we know the rabbit trails that young love and emotional inexperience can lead them down. So Parents often set boundaries for their own children to protect them. Like curfews or no doors closed while in each other's rooms.

Set boundaries for yourself in life too. If you LOVE volunteer work but often find yourself over committing and stretching yourself too thin, set a limit on the number of commitments you make each month. If you love snacking at night set limits on the times you snack and the foods you choose to snack on.

DO NOT set your boundaries too small to start out with. Over time if you're enjoying the freedom that your boundaries are bringing you and want to tighten it up that's fine and if you do set your boundaries too restrictive at first don't feel like you are. Admit right now that's not something I'm able to do and take a step back and yrtagain with some looser boundaries.

I'll use my real life example. Late night snacking. I developed a habit of eating powerballs at night. While filled with a ton of nutrition they are calorie dense and don't fit in when my goals are to cut weight. When I set a boundary of no powerballs ever that's too restrictive makes me feel like I'm missing out on something I enjoy in life. But a boundary of no powerballs after 8pm allows me to keep my favorite treat in my life while cutting back on the amounts I'm eating because I'm less likely to binge during daylight hours. I could then over time also set a limit on the number of times I enjoy my powerball treats a week.

Today's challenge is to identify an area that you feel you could benefit in if you were to set a boundary. If possible break your boundary down into phases like in my example above to make it easier and more likely you'll be able to follow the boundaries you set for yourself over time.

Unit 26

Identify Areas of Improvement

Successful people know how to take constructive criticisms. When we are given feedback we need to evaluate the information honestly and with an open mind. Often we fear criticism. We associate it with imperfection or not being good enough. But the honest truth is we all should be open to criticism because none of us are perfect. We can all improve in some areas of our life.

While we should never talk negatively about ourselves we should be constructively critical of ourselves the same way we would be of a new employee. If we dont direct them in what they should be focusing on improving they simply may not know they need to improve in that area.

Today view yourself as an employee of yourself. Have you been putting in the work? Whatever your goals are, have you been keeping up with them? What do you think you could improve on to help you better or faster reach your goals?

Once you've identified What areas to improve on you can then ask yourself how? How do you improve? You practice! Set smaller goals. Do more research. Keep going!

Life isn't a race it's a journey. When we get to our destination we were done here. PERIOD. Like done. done. Enjoy the journey and don't race to the finish line. Enjoy the adventures and challenges in life because if we are still here. If you woke up today you still have choices to make. Those choices are entirely up to you. It's those choices that are going to take you places. It's up to you which places you want to go.

Unit 27

Gratitude
You don't have to be religious or spiritual to be grateful. Growing up in life I was the type of person to would have complained about having to pay taxes on lottery winnings. Ever watch the shows about how the lottery ruined a life? A show about people that won millions of dollars and then

complained about what happened to them. Ever notice most of the time it was their choices that THEY made that landed them in hot water?

Life doesn't happen to you, it just happens. It's how we react to it that makes the difference in our life. We are all born with blood in our veins. There's no guarantees. There are no givens. Some of us come home to wealthy loving homes. Some of us are born into poverty and abuse. Some of our families are influential. Some of our families are toxic. Some of us experience privilege while others are at a disadvantage. Some people live to see their 100th birthday and some people don't. That's life. It's not always fair and it's not always pretty. But have you ever seen someone coming from a situation that just seems so impossible to recover from one of those heartbroken i feel so lucky right now stories. And they are HAPPY they are grateful they are just impossibly stronger for the experiences. Oftentimes experiencing our lowest lows really show us how high our highs are in life.

Today's challenge is to start a gratitude journal and write down 3 things everyday you are grateful for that aren't food. Really think about all the things going on in your life that you really appreciate. I call them blessings. Even when things seem so low and everything feels like it's falling apart, keeping a positive mind and actively seeking to identify what is going right will help train your brain to continue to look for the good instead of hyper focusing on your problems all the time and compounding our troubles.

Three things I'm grateful for today are: Experiencing Freedom, Having the Opportunity to become a mother and experiencing that one of a kind love, Friendships that I've acquired and learned from.

Unit 28

Your Time is valuable
How much would you pay to spend another hour with a close loved one that's passed away. How much do you make per hour at work? Our time here on this earth is limited. When you are at work your boss decides how much your time is worth. You might be worth $7 an hour to him or $20 an hour to someone else. It's up to you to determine how much your time is worth. Is your time worth spending on facebook and watching tv or is your time better spent on a hobby or playing with your kids. Don't let your time slip away. Every second here on this earth brings you closer to the day you die. It's a fact. How we spend our time can quickly get away from us if we aren't tracking where we are spending it. If you work 48 hrs a week you have left with 5 days of time for yourself, your friends and your family. Ideally a good portion of that will be spent sleeping and resting and the rest is up to you on how you want to spend it. Today's challenge is to begin tracking what you're spending time on and identify if that's really the best use of your time. Are their ways to multitask and save time like doing laundry while cooking dinner? Or maybe you want to start finding ways to work in new hobbies or personal development so you make a sacrifice to get up an extra 30 min earlier each morning to fit in a few hours each week improving your knowledge and skills so you can find a new job and earn more money. Or maybe start a side hustle that you can work while watching tv and walking on an aerobic step.

It's your time you choose how you want to spend it but make sure you're happy with the choices YOU are making!

Unit 29

Keep your promises: To yourself and others. You have friend who says they are meeting you for coffee every saturday for a month and every single time they cancel right before your appointment. Pretty soon you just come to expect them to flake out on you and begin to make other plans. If we make promises we dont keep over and over again we can become that unreliable friend that we say we are going to meet up with but never do. If you make a promise to yourself make sure you are keeping it. We wouldn't make a promise to our boss and then blow off the task and expect no repercussions from it. Just because it's easy to blow off the things we originally wanted to do because something else more pressing came up, don't do it. Over time we become less and less reliable. We expect less and less of ourselves. Today's challenge is to start keeping the promises we are making to ourselves. If someone wants you to sign up for a 30 1 hr workout plan that sounds fun but we are not sure we have the time then be upfront and let them know hey I'm not sure I can prioritize that in my schedule right now maybe another time. Its ok to say no. Just like it's ok for us to set realistic expectations of ourselves. If you're only able to keep a 10 min commitment make a 10 min commitment not a 20 min one.

Unit 30
Use the tools you have available. The rock has a multi thousand dollar gym he brings with him wherever he goes. I'm

not the rock. You're not the rock. So don't expect to have all the tools the rock does have. But we can still get good results without having all the same tools. Maybe you have a sledge hammer and a tire. Use it. Maybe you have your phone and an able body in your living room. Use it. Use what you have around you to help you reach your goals. If you need to use heavy books and canned green beans to work your muscles do it! This unit ties in heavily with becoming an i can person. Look for what you have available to you to help you work towards your goals. If all you can afford is free online videos use those. Today's challenge is to find someone in an adverse position that used an out of the box tool to help them reach their goals. Come back and tell me what you learned through their story and how you plan on using the tools you already have to help yourself towards your goals.

Made in the USA
Coppell, TX
31 October 2021